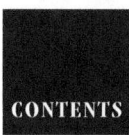

CONTENTS

I0448700

Tables

Figures

Box

Summary

It is frequently stated that about 40 million Americans lack health insurance.[1] That estimate, however, overstates the number of people who are uninsured all year. The Congressional Budget Office (CBO) estimates that between 21 million and 31 million people were uninsured for the entire year in 1998—the most recent year for which reliable comparative data are available. Since then, the number who are uninsured all year probably has not changed substantially, given historical trends. The uninsured population is fluid, with many people gaining and losing coverage. For example, between half and two-thirds of the people who experienced a period of time without insurance in 1998 had coverage for other portions of the year.

The commonly cited estimate of 40 million uninsured comes from the Census Bureau's Current Population Survey (CPS). Based on a large nationally representative sample, the CPS has been collecting data on health insurance status since 1980.

Although the CPS is intended to measure the number of people who lack health coverage for a whole year, its estimate more closely approximates the number of people who are uninsured at a specific point in time during the year. Data from three federally sponsored national surveys—the Survey of Income and Program Participation

(SIPP), the Medical Expenditure Panel Survey (MEPS), and the National Health Interview Survey (NHIS)—yield estimates of the number of uninsured at a particular point in time that are very similar to the CPS estimate of about 40 million (*see Summary Figure 1*). In contrast, data from

Summary Figure 1.

Estimated Number of Nonelderly People Without Health Insurance in 1998

(In millions)

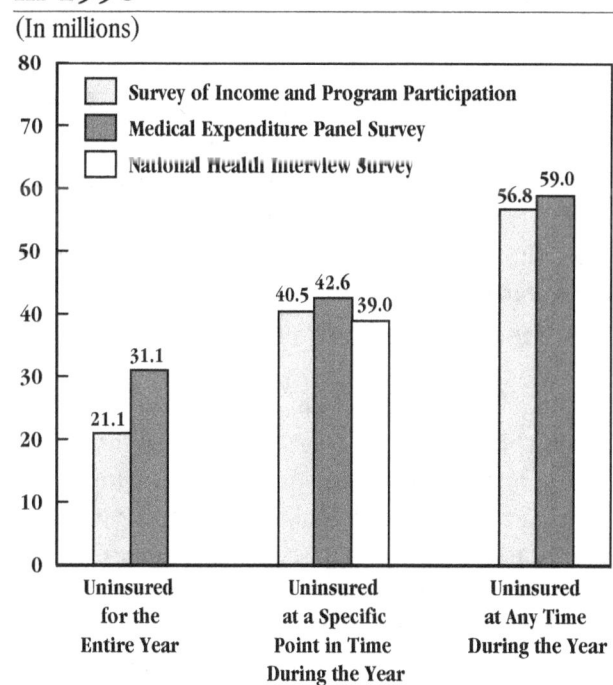

Source: Congressional Budget Office.

Note: The Centers for Disease Control and Prevention, which sponsors the NHIS, reports only the point-in-time estimate.

---

1. See, for example, John M. Broder, "Problem of Lost Health Benefits Is Reaching Into the Middle Class," *New York Times*, November 25, 2002, p. A1; and David Wessel, "The 39 Million Who Mustn't Get Sick," *Wall Street Journal*, December 27, 2001, p. A1.

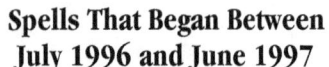

Summary Figure 2.

Distribution of Uninsured Spells Among Nonelderly People in a Given Year and at a Given Point in Time, by Duration

Spells That Began Between July 1996 and June 1997

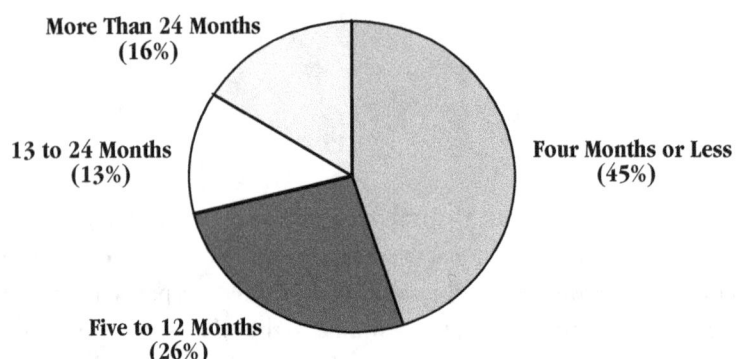

Spells in Progress in March 1998

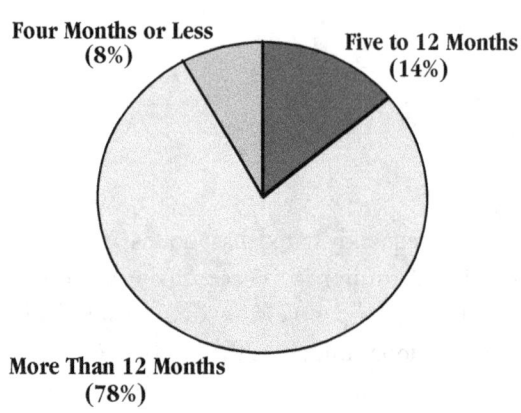

Source: Congressional Budget Office based on data from the first 11 waves of the 1996 panel of the Survey of Income and Program Participation, which followed respondents over a period of 41 months (from March 1996 through July 1999).

SIPP and MEPS indicate that 21 million to 31 million people are uninsured for an entire year.

A third measure of the uninsured is the number of people who lack insurance *at any time* during the year. At nearly 60 million, that measure comprises people who are uninsured for only part of the year and those who are uninsured throughout the year. Together, those three measures of the uninsured provide a more complete picture of that population than any single measure could.

Far from being a static group, the uninsured population is constantly changing. Some people are uninsured for long periods, but more are without coverage for shorter times, such as between jobs. For example, about 30 percent of nonelderly people who become uninsured in a given year remain so for more than 12 months, whereas nearly 50 percent regain health insurance within four months (*see Summary Figure 2*). However, about 80 percent of the people who lack health insurance at a particular time end up being uninsured for more than 12 months. Although long uninsured spells occur less frequently than short spells, they are more likely to be under way at any given time.

Policies aimed at increasing coverage are most likely to be effective if they consider the distinction between the short-term and long-term uninsured. For people with short uninsured spells, policies might have the goal of filling a temporary gap in coverage or of preventing a gap from occurring. For people with longer periods without insurance, policies might seek to provide or facilitate an ongoing source of coverage.

Several sources of uncertainty apply to estimates of the uninsured. Because the estimates come from population surveys, they are prone to reporting error and other forms of statistical error, which could lead to either an underestimate or an overestimate of the size of the uninsured population. For example, underrepresentation of certain segments of the population that are more likely to be uninsured could lead to an undercount of the number of uninsured Americans. Survey estimates could also overstate the number of people who are uninsured, however.

On the basis of comparisons with administrative data, analysts know that fewer people say they have Medicaid coverage than actually do. But some evidence, albeit limited, indicates that many of the Medicaid enrollees who do not report being covered by that program mistakenly report another type of insurance coverage, so that source of bias may be small.

Finally, the concept of insurance and its implications for access to health care are ambiguous in some respects. For example, some people who are counted among the uninsured are eligible for Medicaid. Some policymakers and analysts believe that such people should be regarded as insured, because they can apply for Medicaid when they require care and receive retroactive coverage for their expenses. Others believe that such people should be regarded as uninsured, however, because they do not use Medicaid for their routine medical care (perhaps because they are not aware that they are eligible). Moreover, although a lack of insurance could lead to insufficient access to medical care and exposure to significant financial risk, many people without insurance have access to at least some sources of health care, either through public hospitals, community health centers, local health departments, or Department of Veterans Affairs facilities.

How Many People Lack Health Insurance and For How Long?

More than 240 million people in the United States have health insurance coverage today, through a variety of sources. The vast majority—about 63 percent —are covered through their, or a family member's, employer.[1] Government programs provide coverage to millions more people: about 14 percent have coverage through Medicare, 11 percent through Medicaid and the State Children's Health Insurance Program (SCHIP), and about 3 percent through military programs. Roughly 8 percent of people purchase coverage from private individual health insurers.[2]

Yet millions of people do not have health insurance coverage. For those people, extended periods without insurance could lead to insufficient access to medical care and exposure to significant financial risk. From a broader perspective, a lack of coverage could lead to less efficient use of health care services and facilities, including emergency rooms, and to higher public spending for health programs.

Policymakers have proposed alternatives for expanding health insurance coverage, including providing tax inducements to individuals or employers, expanding Med-

icaid and SCHIP, reforming rules regulating private insurance, and requiring employers to offer coverage.[3] Designing cost-effective policies to expand health coverage requires information on the size and characteristics of the uninsured population. Because many people gain and lose coverage over time, an important feature of uninsured spells is their duration.

This paper presents estimates of the size, demographic characteristics, and dynamics of the uninsured population, using data from four federally sponsored national surveys: the Current Population Survey (CPS), the Survey of Income and Program Participation (SIPP), the Medical Expenditure Panel Survey (MEPS), and the National Health Interview Survey (NHIS). Both the CPS and SIPP are sponsored by the Census Bureau, MEPS by the Agency for Healthcare Research and Quality, and NHIS by the Centers for Disease Control and Prevention. Each survey's strengths and limitations are described in Appendix A.

The Congressional Budget Office's (CBO's) analysis focuses on the nonelderly population because nearly all Americans age 65 and older are covered by Medicare. It excludes people in institutions (such as nursing homes and prisons) because they are not counted in the surveys. Active-duty military personnel are not included in the CPS, MEPS, and NHIS and thus are excluded from CBO's analysis of the data in those surveys, but the analy-

---

1. The federal government exempts employment-based health insurance, among other noncash benefits, from taxation, providing an incentive for the provision of employment-based insurance.

2. See Bureau of the Census, *Health Insurance Coverage: 2001*, Current Population Reports, Series P60-220 (September 2002). The estimates, based on self-reported data from the civilian noninstitutionalized population, are not mutually exclusive; people can be covered by more than one type of insurance in a year.

3. For a discussion of policy options for expanding health insurance coverage, see Congressional Budget Office, *Budget Options* (February 2001), pp. 40-52.

sis of SIPP includes active-duty military personnel, who are counted unless they live in military barracks.

Size of the Uninsured Population

In recent years, the number of uninsured people in the United States has been pegged at approximately 40 million, or about 16 percent of the nonelderly population. By CBO's analysis, that estimate overstates the number of people who are uninsured all year and more closely approximates the number who are uninsured at a point in time during the year. A more accurate estimate of the number of people who were uninsured for all of 1998—the most recent year for which reliable comparative data are available—is 21 million to 31 million, or 9 percent to 13 percent of nonelderly Americans.

The CPS is the source of that widely cited estimate of about 40 million uninsured. By interviewing people in March about their insurance coverage the previous calendar year, the CPS is intended to yield an estimate of the number of people who are uninsured all year. However, comparisons with estimates from other surveys indicate that the CPS estimate overstates that number. Some analysts believe the overstatement stems from an under-reporting of insurance coverage by CPS respondents, who are asked to recall their coverage over a longer period than other surveys require.[4] Other analysts have concluded that the similarity of the CPS estimates to the point-in-time estimates from other surveys suggests that many CPS respondents report their insurance status as of the time of the interview rather than for the previous calendar year, as requested.[5]

In this paper, CBO uses three measures—the number of people who are continuously uninsured for an entire year,

the number who are uninsured at any time during the year, and the number who are uninsured at a point in time—to gauge the size of the uninsured population. Because estimates based on the first two measures use survey data in which people are asked to remember their insurance coverage over a specified period, those data are more prone to reporting error. Point-in-time estimates are subject to less error because people are asked to report their insurance coverage at the time of the interview; however, those estimates do not distinguish between people who are uninsured for a long time and other uninsured people, and they do not reveal how fluid the uninsured population is. Together, the three ways of measuring the uninsured population give a more complete picture than any single measure could.

The Number of People Who Are Uninsured All Year

CBO estimated the number of people who are uninsured all year using data from SIPP and MEPS, two surveys in which respondents are interviewed multiple times over the life of the survey. (Such longitudinal surveys allow researchers to repeatedly observe a set of subjects over time.) SIPP interviews people every four months about their insurance coverage during the preceding four months (called a "wave"), while MEPS interviews people every four to five months, on average. By asking people to remember their insurance status over a shorter period of time than the CPS requires, SIPP and MEPS should yield more accurate estimates of the number of people who are uninsured all year.[6]

According to the most recent SIPP data, 9.1 percent of the nonelderly population (or 21.1 million people) were continuously uninsured throughout 1998 (see Table 1).[7] According to MEPS, the corresponding figures were 13.3 percent (or 31.1 million people). The discrepancy between those estimates could be due to various factors, including differences in the wording and sequencing of

4. Robert L. Bennefield, "A Comparative Analysis of Health Insurance Coverage Estimates: Data from CPS and SIPP" (paper presented at the Joint Statistical Meetings, American Statistical Association, Chicago, Ill., August 6, 1996).

5. Katherine Swartz, "Interpreting the Estimates from Four National Surveys of the Number of People Without Health Insurance," *Journal of Economic and Social Measurement*, vol. 14 (1986), pp. 233-242.

6. SIPP and MEPS also have certain limitations, which are discussed in Appendix A.

7. These figures are based on analysis of data from the 1996 panel of the Survey of Income and Program Participation, which followed all respondents through July 1999. Because only a limited amount of data from the 2001 SIPP is now available, CBO's analysis does not rely on that version of the survey.

Table 1.

Percentage and Number of Nonelderly People Without Health Insurance in 1998 and 1999, Estimated from Four National Surveys

| | Uninsured Nonelderly People | | | |
| | In percent | | In millions | |
	1998	1999	1998	1999
Uninsured All Year				
SIPP	9.1	n.a.	21.1	n.a.
MEPS	13.3	12.2	31.1	28.9
Uninsured at Any Time During the Year				
SIPP	24.5	n.a.	56.8	n.a.
MEPS	25.3	25.1	59.0	59.2
Uninsured at a Point in Time				
SIPP	16.6	15.7	40.5	38.5
MEPS	18.3	17.4	42.6	41.0
NHIS	16.5	16.0	39.0	38.3
CPS[a]	18.4	16.2	43.9	39.0

Source: Congressional Budget Office based on data from the 1996 panel of the Survey of Income and Program Participation (SIPP), the 1998 and 1999 Medical Expenditure Panel Survey (MEPS), and the March 1999 and March 2000 Current Population Survey (CPS). Estimates from the National Health Interview Survey (NHIS) are from the Centers for Disease Control and Prevention, "Early Release of Selected Estimates Based on Data from the 2001 NHIS," available at www.cdc.gov/nchs.

Note: n.a. = not available.

a. The CPS estimate is intended to measure the number of people who are uninsured for the entire year. However, there is considerable evidence that the CPS estimate overstates the number of people who are uninsured all year and is closer to the number of people who are uninsured at a point in time. About two-thirds of the reduction in the CPS estimate of the number of uninsured from 1998 to 1999 was due to the inclusion of an additional question in the survey that was designed to yield more-accurate estimates.

questions on health insurance coverage, data editing procedures, interviewers' training and knowledge about health insurance, and the period of time over which people were asked to recall their coverage.

Data from MEPS also indicate that the number of people who were uninsured all year fell from 31.1 million in 1998 to 28.9 million in 1999 (estimates from MEPS of the full-year uninsured are not available for more recent years). But recent trends in the CPS estimates—which are similar to the point-in-time estimates from SIPP, MEPS, and NHIS—suggest that the number of people who were uninsured all year probably remained relatively stable from 1999 to 2000 and then increased somewhat in

2001.[8] That conclusion is based on the fact that the full-year and point-in-time estimates of the uninsured are likely to move in a similar manner over time. More recently, the number who are uninsured all year probably has not changed substantially, given historical trends.

The Number of People Who Are Uninsured at Any Time During the Year

CBO's analysis of data from SIPP and MEPS indicates that about a quarter of the nonelderly population (or

---

8. According to the CPS, the number of nonelderly people who lacked health insurance rose from 39.6 million in 2000 to 40.9 million in 2001, after falling slightly the previous year.

about 57 million to 59 million Americans) was uninsured at any time during 1998 (see Table 1). According to MEPS, that measure remained essentially unchanged from 1998 to 1999. If the elderly were included in the analysis, the percentage of the population that was uninsured at any time during the year would have fallen to 22 percent.[9]

Analysis of SIPP and MEPS data also shows that the uninsured population is very fluid. According to data from SIPP, roughly 63 percent of the people who were uninsured at any time in 1998 lost coverage or gained coverage (or did both) at some point during the year.[10] The corresponding figure from MEPS was 47 percent, increasing to 51 percent in 1999.

The Number of People Who Are Uninsured at a Point in Time

Data from SIPP, MEPS, and NHIS yield similar estimates of the number of people who are uninsured at a given point in time.[11] The point-in-time estimates from those surveys, which are very similar to the CPS estimates, ranged from 39.0 million to 42.6 million uninsured in 1998, or from 16.5 percent to 18.3 percent of the nonelderly population (see Table 1). That range of

estimates fell slightly in 1999, according to all four surveys. Taken altogether, the point-in-time estimates from SIPP, MEPS, and NHIS provide compelling evidence that the CPS overstates the number of people who are uninsured all year.

Although analyses of the uninsured typically focus on individual-level data, analyses at the family level provide a measure of the total number of families that are potential targets of policymakers' efforts to expand coverage. According to data from SIPP, approximately 26 million families had at least one person who was uninsured at a given point in time in 1998.[12] In 27 percent of those families, however, at least one person was insured. Such families represent a variety of circumstances, including those in which children are covered under Medicaid or SCHIP but parents are not or only some members are covered by an employment-based (or private nongroup) policy.

The relationship between the number of people who are uninsured at a particular point in time and the number who are uninsured all year appears to have not changed significantly—at least since 1992—although the evidence supporting that conclusion is limited. The most direct comparison of the two measures comes from a study of SIPP data that found that 14.8 percent of Americans (including the elderly) were uninsured at a point in time in 1992, while 7.6 percent were uninsured all year.[13] That nearly two-to-one ratio is echoed in the 1998 figures from SIPP, 16.6 percent versus 9.1 percent. Indirect evidence that a similar relationship probably held in earlier years comes from studies (discussed below) showing that the duration of uninsured spells among the nonelderly population had a distribution similar to that found in this analysis.

---

9. Including military personnel and the institutionalized—all of whom are either insured or have access to medical care—would also reduce the percentage of the population that was uninsured at any time during the year, but by a much smaller amount than would be obtained by including the elderly. The magnitude of the reduction cannot be determined from available data; information is not available on the insurance status of people who spend part of a year in the military or an institution. However, such an analysis is possible when measuring insurance coverage at a point in time. Using data from SIPP, CBO estimates that including the military and the institutionalized in the analysis would reduce the percentage of nonelderly who were uninsured at a point in time in 1999 by about 0.1 percentage point.

10. Some 15.4 percent of the nonelderly population was uninsured for part, but not all, of 1998. Such people constitute 62.9 percent of the total nonelderly population that was uninsured at any time in 1998.

11. NHIS estimates are from Centers for Disease Control and Prevention, National Center for Health Statistics, "Early Release of Selected Estimates Based on Data from the 2001 NHIS" (released July 15, 2002).

12. Families are defined in this analysis as health insurance eligibility units, on the basis of eligibility rules of most private insurance plans. In households with two or more people, those rules were applied to identify all individuals who would be eligible for coverage under a family policy. This definition of families also includes single adults.

13. Bennefield, "A Comparative Analysis of Health Insurance Coverage Estimates."

The Implications of the Medicaid Undercount

The number of people who report that they have Medicaid coverage in population surveys is smaller than the number indicated by the program's administrative data. Less clear than the fact of the undercount itself, however, are its size and its implications for estimates of the uninsured.

Underreporting of Medicaid coverage could occur for various reasons. Some people might not report their coverage in a survey because of the stigma associated with participating in a public assistance program. Also, some people covered by Medicaid may mistakenly believe that they have another type of coverage, such as private insurance. That confusion may be most common among people enrolled in Medicaid managed care because such programs often use names designated by private plans or by a state's Medicaid agency that do not include the term "Medicaid."

According to one study, SIPP undercounts Medicaid enrollment relative to the administrative data maintained by the Centers for Medicare and Medicaid Services by about 12 percent to 15 percent.[14] CBO's analysis of data from MEPS indicates that that survey undercounts Medicaid enrollment by a similar amount. Those findings may imply that the number of nonelderly people who are enrolled in Medicaid at any time during the year could be undercounted in population surveys by about 4 million to 5 million.

Estimates of the size of the Medicaid undercount must be viewed with caution, however, because of limitations of the administrative data that are used as the benchmark.[15] Even if those estimates are correct, they do not necessarily imply a corresponding error in the count of the uninsured, because some Medicaid enrollees who do not report having Medicaid coverage may report another type of coverage. One study that matched Medicaid administrative records in Minnesota with a population survey conducted in that state found that the vast majority of Medicaid enrollees who did not report being covered by Medicaid reported another source of insurance.[16] As a result, the measured uninsurance rate was overstated by only about 0.3 percentage points. It is not known how those findings may be generalized to other states or other surveys.

Because of uncertainties about the size of the Medicaid undercount and its implications for estimates of the uninsured, CBO did not adjust its analysis to compensate for the undercount.

The Implications of Less-Than-Full Participation in Medicaid

Many people who are eligible for Medicaid do not participate in the program. Research estimates that about half of eligible nonparticipants have private coverage and half are uninsured.[17] For uninsured people who are eligible but not enrolled, Medicaid provides a form of conditional coverage. Such people can apply for Medicaid at the time they obtain care and receive retroactive coverage for their expenses.[18] Because of that provision, some policymakers view those people as insured. Others view them as uninsured because they may not realize that they are eligible for Medicaid and therefore may delay or avoid seeking medical care.

An estimated 2.9 million children were uninsured but eligible for Medicaid at a given point in time in 1994 (the most recent year for which estimates are available). That figure represents about one-third of uninsured children

---

14. John L. Czajka, *Analysis of Children's Health Insurance Patterns: Findings from the SIPP* (report submitted by Mathematica Policy Research, Inc., to the Department of Health and Human Services, Assistant Secretary for Planning and Evaluation, May 1999).

15. The administrative data maintained by the Centers for Medicare and Medicaid Services are reported separately by each state and are subject to reporting errors. The "ever enrolled" estimates are intended to represent an unduplicated count of the number of people enrolled in Medicaid at any time during the fiscal year.

16. Kathleen Thiede Call and others, "Uncovering the Missing Medicaid Cases and Assessing Their Bias for Estimates of the Uninsured," *Inquiry*, vol. 38, no. 4 (Winter 2001/2002), pp. 396-408.

17. All estimates reported in this section are from Czajka, *Analysis of Children's Health Insurance Patterns.*

18. Jonathan Gruber, *Medicaid*, Working Paper No. 7829 (Cambridge, Mass: National Bureau of Economic Research, August 2000).

and about 17 percent of all children who were eligible for Medicaid. For many children, being eligible for Medicaid while uninsured is a short-term phenomenon. Many such children are in transition from one source of coverage to another (for example, from private insurance to Medicaid), and others are eligible for Medicaid for a short period because of a temporary decline in family income. Even so, an estimated 1 million children remained uninsured all year in 1994 even though they were eligible for Medicaid.

Demographic Characteristics of the Uninsured Population

Education and income level are closely tied to the likelihood of being uninsured. According to data from SIPP, 25 percent of people in families in which no one had a high school diploma were uninsured all year in 1998, and 50 percent were uninsured at any time during the year (*see Table 2*). Similar percentages of people in families with income below 200 percent of the poverty level were uninsured in 1998. Hispanics had a higher rate of being uninsured all year in 1998 than other racial and ethnic groups (23 percent), and young adults ages 19 to 24 were more likely than people in other age groups to be uninsured all year (14 percent).

The likelihood of being uninsured does not vary greatly by self-reported health status. According to SIPP data, about 10 percent of people who said they were in poor health were uninsured all year in 1998; that figure is similar to the percentages of people in excellent or very good health who lacked insurance coverage all year.[19] Because individuals in poor health constitute a relatively small proportion of the total nonelderly population, they accounted for only 5 percent of the full-year uninsured in 1998. As a group, however, they may be of particular concern to policymakers because they are likely to be the greatest users of health care services.

Nearly 90 percent of the people who were uninsured all year in 1998 were in families in which at least one person

worked, either part time or full time (*see Table 2, column 3*). Research has found that about 75 percent of the uninsured in working families do not have access to insurance through their employer, the dominant form of coverage among the nonelderly, while the other 25 percent have access to employment-based insurance but do not accept it.[20] Lower-wage workers are less likely than higher earners to have access to employment-based insurance and are less likely to accept it where it is offered.[21]

Dynamics of the Uninsured Population

CBO's analysis of SIPP data reveals that although many uninsured spells are relatively short, some are quite long. Many people who become uninsured are in transition from one source of coverage to another (for example, because of a waiting period for coverage at a new job), so their uninsured spells are relatively brief.

The Duration of Uninsured Spells

CBO measured the duration of uninsured spells in two ways. First, it estimated the duration of spells that began during the 12-month period from July 1996 through June 1997.[22] Because new spells closely approximate a representative sample of all uninsured spells, they provide the most reliable basis for estimating durations.[23] Second, because policy discussions often refer to the uninsured

---

19. Information on health status was collected in interviews between August 1997 and November 1997. Survey respondents were at least 15 years of age.

20. Sherry Glied, "Challenges and Options for Increasing the Number of Americans with Health Insurance," *Inquiry*, vol. 38, no. 2 (Summer 2001), pp. 90-105.

21. Philip F. Cooper and Barbara Steinberg Schone, "More Offers, Fewer Takers for Employment-Based Health Insurance: 1987 and 1996," *Health Affairs*, vol.16, no. 6 (November/December 1997), pp.142-149.

22. CBO also estimated the duration of uninsured spells that began during other periods—for example, during each month within the July 1996-June 1997 period and during the 24-month span from July 1996 through June 1998. Similar results were obtained for all of those periods.

23. Katherine Swartz, John Marcotte, and Timothy D. McBride, "Spells Without Health Insurance: The Distribution of Durations When Left-Censored Spells Are Included," *Inquiry*, vol. 30 (Spring 1993), pp. 77-83.

Table 2.

Nonelderly People Without Health Insurance in 1998, by Selected Characteristics

(In percent)

Characteristic	Nonelderly People		Distribution of the Population Uninsured All Year
	Uninsured at Any Time During the Year	Uninsured All Year	
Age			
Less than 19	26.8	7.3	24.9
19 to 24	41.9	14.4	13.7
25 to 34	31.1	12.3	21.9
35 to 44	20.2	9.3	19.7
45 to 54	15.1	7.6	12.6
55 to 64	14.0	6.7	7.2
Race/Ethnicity			
White, Non-Hispanic	18.4	6.3	48.4
Black, Non-Hispanic	33.4	10.7	15.3
Hispanic	47.4	22.5	30.8
Other	31.1	10.9	5.5
Family Income Relative to the Poverty Level[a]			
Less than 200 percent	47.9	19.5	74.9
200 percent to 399 percent	17.4	5.3	19.8
400 percent or more	6.0	1.6	5.3
Education[a,b]			
No high school diploma	50.4	24.6	28.4
High school graduate	33.1	12.7	36.4
Some college coursework	22.1	7.3	26.6
Bachelor's degree or higher	9.9	2.6	8.7
Family Employment Status[a]			
At least one full-time worker all year	15.0	5.9	42.9
Part-time or part-year work only	46.1	16.1	46.6
No work	32.8	13.1	10.6
Health Status[c]			
Excellent	23.7	8.9	28.8
Very good	25.1	9.3	32.8
Good	24.6	9.1	24.5
Fair	25.1	8.7	8.9
Poor	25.3	10.3	5.1
Memorandum:			
Total Nonelderly Population	24.5	9.1	100.0

Source: Congressional Budget Office based on data from the 1996 panel of the Survey of Income and Program Participation.

a. For family-level variables, families are defined as health insurance eligibility units, which are composed of individuals who could be covered as a family under most private health insurance plans.

b. Education is defined as the highest education level among all adults in the family.

c. Information on health status was collected only for survey respondents who were at least 15 years of age.

Box 1.

Two Approaches to Measuring Uninsured Spells

Consider five people who become uninsured at some time during a year. Person A becomes uninsured in January and is uninsured for the entire year. The other four people are each uninsured for three months, the first from January through March, the second from April through June, and so on (*see figure, below*). If the duration of uninsured spells is measured by including all spells that begin during the year, 20 percent (one of five) last 12 months and 80 percent (four of five) last three months. If, instead, durations are measured by including only spells that are in progress at a particular point in time, 50 percent (one of two) last 12 months and 50 percent last three months. The first approach measures the duration of all uninsured spells that begin during the year, while the second approach characterizes spells at a given point in time.

Duration of Uninsured Spells

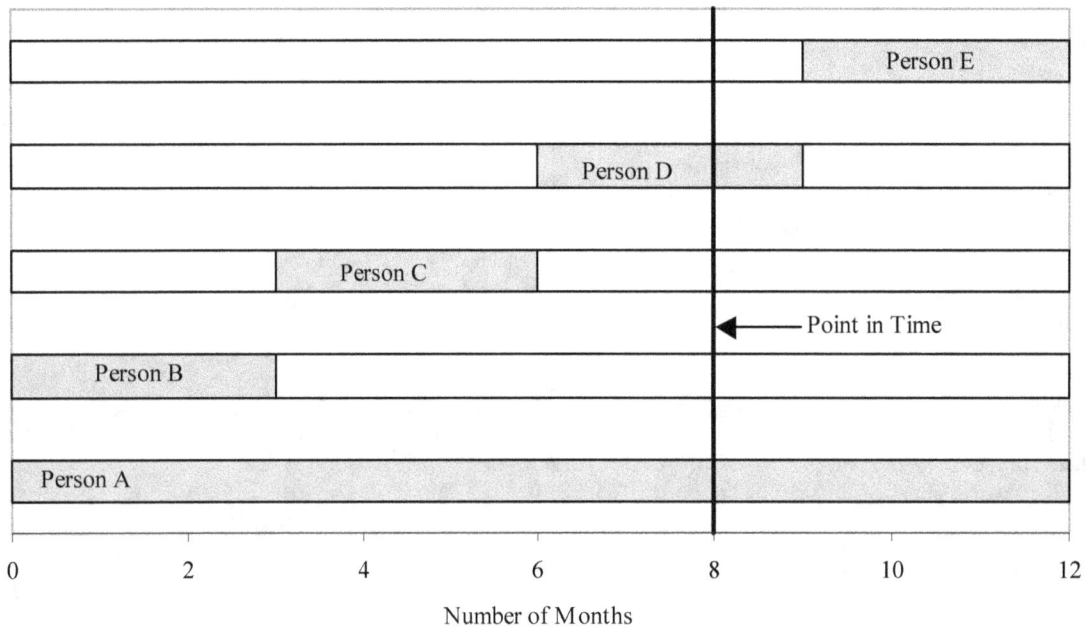

Number of Months

---

population at a given point in time, CBO estimated the duration of spells among people who were uninsured in a given month. The first measure captures the *flow* of uninsured spells over time, while the second captures the *stock* of uninsured spells at a point in time. The two measures yield very different estimates of durations (*see Box 1*).

New Spells. Forty-five percent of the uninsured spells that began between July 1996 and June 1997 lasted four months or less, whereas about 16 percent lasted more than 24 months (*see the top panel of Table 3*). Those figures correspond to estimates obtained by other researchers using SIPP data from 1983 to 1986 and 1992 to 1994.[24] Children under 19 were more likely than

---

24. Katherine Swartz and Timothy D. McBride, "Spells Without Health Insurance: Distributions of Durations and Their Link to Point-in-Time Estimates of the Uninsured," *Inquiry*, vol. 27 (Fall 1990), pp. 281-288; and Czajka, *Analysis of Children's Health Insurance Patterns*. The unemployment rate was much higher during the years covered by those studies, indicating that the duration of uninsured spells has not varied much with changes in economic conditions.

Table 3.

Distribution of Uninsured Spells by Duration and Age

(In percent)

Duration of Uninsured Spell	Total Nonelderly Population	Children	Adults
Spells That Began Between July 1996 and June 1997			
Four Months or Less	44.5	49.3	41.0
Five to 12 Months	26.2	25.2	26.9
13 to 24 Months	13.4	11.8	14.5
More Than 24 Months	15.9	13.7	17.6
Spells in Progress in March 1998[a]			
Four Months or Less	7.9	12.9	5.6
Five to 12 Months	14.4	19.3	12.3
More Than 12 Months	77.8	67.8	82.0

Source: Congressional Budget Office based on data from the 1996 panel of the Survey of Income and Program Participation.

Notes: Children are defined as people under 19 years of age, adults as people ages 19 through 64.

Appendix B explains the consistency of the two sets of estimates given in this table.

a.   The estimates for spells in progress in March 1998 measure the total duration of such spells, looking backward and forward in time (the observation period extended through July 1999). Similar estimates were obtained for other months.

adults to have short uninsured spells. Forty-nine percent of the spells experienced by children lasted four months or less, compared with 41 percent for adults.

A potential limitation of measuring durations from a sample of new spells is that people who are uninsured for a long time may be underrepresented. By definition, analyses of new spells focus on spells for which a starting point can be observed. Spells that were in progress at the start of SIPP's observation period (so-called left-censored spells) are excluded, so individuals who were uninsured throughout the entire period are excluded from the calculation of durations.[25] Previous research suggests, however, that excluding left-censored spells does not dramatically alter the results of the analysis.[26]

---

25. Four percent of the people in SIPP's sample were uninsured throughout the entire 41-month observation period.

26. See Swartz, Marcotte, and McBride, "Spells Without Health Insurance." Using sophisticated econometric methods in an analysis of data from the 1984 SIPP panel, the authors estimated that including left-censored spells reduced the share of spells that lasted five months or less from 50 percent to 48 percent and increased the share of spells that lasted more than 24 months from 15 percent

Spells in Progress at a Point in Time. Compared with the duration of new spells, the duration of those in progress at a given point in time is much more likely to be relatively long. More than three-quarters of the uninsured spells in progress in March 1998 exceeded 12 months, whereas only about 8 percent lasted four months or less (*see the bottom panel of Table 3*). Those estimates measure the total length of the spells in progress in March 1998, looking backward and forward in time. Similar estimates were obtained for other months.

Although estimates of the duration of new spells and spells in progress in a particular month differ dramatically, they simply represent alternative ways of looking at the uninsured population. Nearly half of all new spells end within four months; over time, as those shorter spells end and longer spells remain in effect, the stock of uninsured spells at a given point in time has a relatively high proportion of long spells. Looked at another way, a par-

---

to 19 percent. The median duration increased from six months to seven months. Those findings indicate that long-term uninsured people are underrepresented among new spells, but not by enough to invalidate the basic conclusions of analyses that focus solely on new spells.

ticular long spell is more likely to be in progress at a given point in time than a particular short spell. (Appendix B demonstrates the consistency of the two sets of estimates in Table 3.) The analysis in the rest of this paper focuses on new spells, because they more accurately represent all uninsured spells.

Characteristics Associated with the Duration of Uninsured Spells

The duration of spells varies with education level, race/ethnicity, and income of the uninsured. People with less education are more likely than higher-educated people to experience long uninsured spells. Some 23 percent of spells among people in families in which no one graduated from high school last more than two years, compared with a figure of only 8 percent among people in families in which at least one person has a bachelor's degree (*see Table 4*). That relationship probably reflects, at least in part, the fact that college-educated people are more likely than those with less education to have access to employment-based insurance.[27] Long uninsured spells are also more common among Hispanics and people with low income.[28] For example, 23 percent of uninsured spells among Hispanics last more than two years, compared with 14 percent of spells among non-Hispanic

whites and 15 percent among non-Hispanic blacks. Eighteen percent of uninsured spells among people with annual income of less than 200 percent of the federal poverty level exceed two years, about two-thirds higher than the figure for people whose income is 400 percent or more of the poverty level.

The duration of uninsured spells does not vary much with self-reported health status. For instance, 14 percent of uninsured spells among people in poor health last more than two years, nearly the same percentage of spells as among people reporting very good health. By keeping some people from working full time, however, poor health may contribute to long uninsured spells. Those spells may be of particular concern from a policy perspective because such people are likely to be intensive users of health care services.

As noted previously, adults are more likely than children to experience long uninsured spells. The availability of Medicaid coverage may explain some of that discrepancy: coverage is available to many children in low-income families, but the great majority of low-income adults are not eligible for the program. In addition, single adults without children may be less inclined to seek insurance, on average, than other adults are, which may lead them to experience long spells without insurance.[29]

Multiple Spells and Total Uninsured Months

While the preceding analysis looked only at people who had one uninsured spell, to obtain a more complete picture of the uninsured this section looks at whether many uninsured people have multiple spells. The subsequent experience of people whose initial uninsured spell was relatively short is of particular interest. Did most of those people have a single uninsured spell? Or did many of them have additional spells, perhaps experiencing substantial periods without coverage?

To investigate those issues, CBO analyzed data from the 1996 SIPP panel, following people who had one unin-

---

27. Higher-wage workers are more likely to be offered employment-based insurance, and wages are highly correlated with education. For evidence of the relationship between wages and the likelihood of being offered employment-based insurance, see Cooper and Schone, "More Offers, Fewer Takers for Employment-Based Health Insurance."

28. For this analysis, family income relative to the poverty level was defined as the mean value during the four months before the uninsured spell began. The intent was to classify families on the basis of their income before they experienced any reduction in income that may have accompanied the uninsured spell. Such an income reduction may have been temporary for many families but longer-lasting for others. The income measure was intended to reflect, for many families, their longer-term economic circumstances. The analysis was also conducted using a second income measure, defined as the mean family income relative to the poverty level during the first four months of the uninsured spell (or during the entire spell if it ended within four months). The second measure captures any changes in families' economic circumstances that occurred around the time the uninsured spell began. Estimates using the second measure (which this paper does not present) are similar to the estimates in Table 4.

29. That conclusion is supported by analysis conducted for this study (but not reported in detail here), which found that after controlling for differences in age, race/ethnicity, education, and income relative to the poverty level, single adults without children were much more likely than other adults to experience long uninsured spells.

Table 4.

Distribution of Uninsured Spells by Duration and Selected Characteristics

(In percent)

Characteristic	Four Months or Less	Five to 12 Months	13 to 24 Months	More Than 24 Months
Age[a]				
Less than 19	49.1	25.4	11.8	13.7
19 to 24	41.1	28.5	16.8	13.6
25 to 34	42.6	26.3	14.2	16.9
35 to 44	40.5	25.6	13.0	20.9
45 to 54	40.4	26.0	13.5	20.1
55 to 64	37.5	28.1	14.4	20.0
Race/Ethnicity				
White, Non-Hispanic	46.9	26.6	12.8	13.8
Black, Non-Hispanic	45.1	27.6	12.3	15.1
Hispanic	39.5	21.4	16.0	23.0
Other	38.9	34.7	12.6	13.8
Family Income Relative to the Poverty Level[b,c]				
Less than 200 percent	41.8	26.1	14.3	17.9
200 percent to 399 percent	47.6	27.7	11.7	13.0
400 percent or more	55.3	22.9	11.1	10.7
Education[a,c]				
No high school diploma	39.0	22.6	15.2	23.2
High school graduate	40.7	26.7	15.8	16.8
Some college coursework	48.3	27.7	10.1	13.9
Bachelor's degree or higher	53.0	26.8	12.3	7.9
Health Status[d]				
Excellent	41.9	26.4	14.1	17.7
Very good	47.5	24.6	13.1	14.8
Good	42.8	29.7	11.6	16.0
Fair	46.1	19.4	12.5	22.0
Poor	46.3	26.8	12.6	14.3
Memorandum:				
Total Nonelderly Population	44.5	26.2	13.4	15.9

Source: Congressional Budget Office based on data from the 1996 panel of the Survey of Income and Program Participation.

Notes: Distributions sum to 100 across rows.

Estimates in this table are based on uninsured spells that began between July 1996 and June 1997.

a. Age and education were measured as of the first month of the uninsured spell. Education is defined as the highest education level among all adults in the family.
b. Family income relative to the poverty level was computed as the mean over the four-month period before the beginning of the uninsured spell. Similar results were obtained when family income relative to the poverty level was defined as the mean during the first four months of the uninsured spell (or during the entire spell if it ended within four months).
c. For family-level variables, families are defined as health insurance eligibility units, which are composed of individuals who could be covered as a family under most private health insurance plans.
d. Information on health status was collected in interviews between August 1997 and November 1997. Survey respondents were at least 15 years of age.

Table 5.

Distribution of Uninsured Spells and Uninsured Months Among Nonelderly People Who Had a Spell That Began Between July 1996 and June 1997

(In percent)

	All Nonelderly People	People with an Initial Spell of	
		Four Months or Less	More Than 12 Months
Adults with Uninsured Spells, by Total Number of Spells			
One Spell	57.7	49.7	78.5
Two Spells	32.3	35.9	19.6
Three Spells	9.0	12.7	1.8
More Than Three Spells	1.0	1.7	0.1
Adults with Uninsured Spells, by Total Number of Months			
Four Months or Less	21.8	49.0	n.a.
Five to 12 Months	27.4	28.4	n.a.
13 to 24 Months	27.0	17.1	35.2
More Than 24 Months	23.7	5.5	64.8

Source: Congressional Budget Office based on data from the 1996 panel of the Survey of Income and Program Participation.

Notes: n.a. = not applicable.

The total number of uninsured spells and insured months covers the period from July 1996 through June 1999.

sured spell that began between July 1996 and June 1997 over the 36-month period ending in June 1999. Just under 60 percent of such people had no additional uninsured spells; 32 percent had one additional spell; and 10 percent had more than one additional spell (*see the first column in Table 5*, which shows the distribution by total number of spells). About 22 percent of the people were uninsured for a total of four months or less during the 36 months examined; nearly one-quarter (23.7 percent) were uninsured for more than 24 months.

About half of the people whose initial uninsured spell ended within four months had at least one additional spell during the 36-month period (*see the second column in Table 5*). More than three-quarters of the people with a short initial spell were uninsured for less than 12 months during the extended 36-month period; only 6 percent were uninsured for more than 24 months.

Reasons Reported for Lacking Health Insurance

The high cost of insurance and lack of access to employment-based coverage are the two most commonly re-

ported reasons for being uninsured. More than 60 percent of uninsured adults cited one or both of those factors as contributing to their lack of coverage (*see Table 6*).[30] Only about 4 percent of nonelderly adults cited poor health as a reason for being uninsured. Although that figure suggests that a relatively small fraction of the uninsured had been denied coverage in the nongroup insurance market because of poor health, some people who cited the high cost of insurance as a reason for being uninsured may have declined coverage in the nongroup market after being "rated up" because of their medical conditions. One percent of uninsured adults indicated that they did not have insurance because they could obtain medical care from a Department of Veterans Affairs (VA) hospital.

People who have been uninsured for more than 12 months are more likely than those who have been uninsured for four months or less to lack coverage because of its high cost (98 percent versus 49 percent), because they do not have access to employment-based coverage

---

30. CBO's analysis was based on SIPP data on adults with an uninsured spell that began between July 1996 and June 1997.

Table 6.

Reasons Reported by Nonelderly Adults for Lacking Health Insurance

(In percent)

	All Nonelderly Adults	Adults with an Uninsured Spell of	
		Four Months or Less	More Than 12 Months
High Cost	71.0	49.4	97.5
Lack of Access to Employer-Sponsored Insurance	61.6	43.8	83.3
Attitudes/Preferences			
Have not needed insurance	9.9	4.3	17.0
Do not believe in insurance	1.0	1.1	1.6
Other			
No longer covered by parents	6.1	4.2	8.8
Poor health	3.5	1.6	6.3
Use VA hospital	1.4	0.4	2.4

Source: Congressional Budget Office based on data from the 1996 panel of the Survey of Income and Program Participation.

Notes: The analysis was based on responses of adults ages 19 through 64 with an uninsured spell that began between July 1996 and June 1997.

Percentages do not sum to 100 because respondents were allowed to give more than one reason.

VA = Department of Veterans Affairs.

(83 percent versus 44 percent), or because they have not needed insurance in the past (17 percent versus 4 percent). Those discrepancies may in part reflect the fact that people who are uninsured for shorter periods may not regard their temporary lack of coverage as a problem. For example, if people's lack of access to employment-based insurance is a temporary phenomenon (for example, because of a change in jobs), they may not report it in a survey. Similarly, many people with relatively short uninsured spells may not cite high cost as a reason for being uninsured because they did not investigate the cost of insurance options (such as private nongroup coverage) to fill the gap in coverage.

Policy Considerations

To expand health insurance coverage, policymakers have proposed various options. They include offering tax inducements for insurance coverage, expanding Medicaid and the State Children's Health Insurance Program, reforming rules regulating private insurance, and requiring employers to offer coverage.

In considering any approach to expand health coverage, policymakers should be mindful of the fact that many people are uninsured for relatively short periods, whereas others are uninsured for much longer spans. Developing policies geared toward the long-term uninsured—the group that some policymakers consider most important—is not straightforward. For example, one might think that a program to expand insurance coverage among low-income people would primarily benefit the long-term uninsured. But CBO's analysis shows that 42 percent of uninsured spells among people with income below 200 percent of the poverty level end within four months, while only about one-third last more than a year.

Another issue that complicates any policy initiative to expand health insurance is the crowding out of existing sources of coverage.[31] "Crowd-out" results when coverage

31. For a review of the literature on crowd-out, see *Understanding the Dynamics of "Crowd-out": Defining Public/Private Coverage Substitution for Policy and Research* (report prepared by the Academy for Health Services Research and Health Policy under The Robert Wood Johnson Foundation's Changes in Health Care Financing and Organization (HCFO) Program, June 2001).

through a new government policy initiative replaces private coverage that people would have otherwise had. Crowd-out can occur in various ways. Some employees may drop their employment-based coverage if a government program provides health insurance at a lower premium. Or employers may reduce or drop coverage if their employees have less demand for such a benefit because a government program provides an alternative source of coverage. A related issue concerns health insurance tax credits. Some proposals for those tax credits would "buy up the base" by extending credits to people who would have been insured even without them. Both phenomena result in federal subsidies being extended to people who otherwise would have been insured. As a result, the federal cost per *newly* insured person could be substantially greater than the cost for each person who uses the federal program or receives the tax credit.

Several sources of uncertainty apply to estimates of the uninsured population. Because the estimates come from population surveys, they are prone to reporting error and other forms of statistical error, which could lead to either an underestimate or an overestimate of the size of the uninsured population. On the one hand, certain segments of the population that are more likely to be uninsured (such as Hispanics) are less likely to be fully represented in those surveys.[32] That underrepresentation could lead

to an undercount of the number of uninsured. On the other hand, to the extent that Medicaid enrollees are incorrectly classified as uninsured, survey estimates overstate the number of people who are uninsured.

Furthermore, the concept of insurance and its implications for access to health care are ambiguous in some respects. Some people who report being uninsured may be eligible for some type of government coverage but are not enrolled. Eligible low-income people can apply for Medicaid when they require care, for example, and receive retroactive coverage for their expenses. For that reason, some policymakers believe such people should be viewed as insured. Others view such people as uninsured, because they do not use Medicaid for their routine medical care (perhaps because they are unaware that they are eligible). Moreover, although a lack of insurance could lead to insufficient access to medical care and exposure to significant financial risk, many people without insurance have access to at least some sources of health care. Safety net providers—such as public hospitals, community health centers, and local health departments—deliver significant amounts of care to people without insurance coverage, and military veterans are eligible to receive care at VA facilities.

---

32. Analysts have studied that phenomenon, which is known as undercoverage. See U.S. Census Bureau and Bureau of Labor Statistics, "Technical Paper 63RV: Current Population Survey—Design and Methodology" (March 2002), available at www.census.gov/prod/2002pubs/tp63rv.pdf.

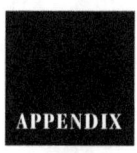

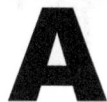

Strengths and Limitations of the Survey Data

The data underlying the analysis in this report come from the Current Population Survey (CPS), the Survey of Income and Program Participation (SIPP), the Medical Expenditure Panel Survey (MEPS), and the National Health Interview Survey (NHIS). All four surveys use large nationally representative samples of the civilian noninstitutionalized population to measure the uninsured. This appendix details each survey's advantages and disadvantages.

The Current Population Survey

The Census Bureau's Current Population Survey is designed to measure the number of people in the United States who are uninsured all year. An important advantage of the CPS is its timely release. Data collected in the March CPS (for the previous calendar year) are typically released six months later, in September. In addition, because of the survey's methodology and sample size, the data can be broken out by state.

The CPS has some limitations, however. First, it has a relatively long reference period for measuring insurance status. That long reference period may partly explain how the CPS estimate overstates the number of people who are uninsured all year. Some analysts have speculated that many CPS respondents report their insurance status as of the time of the interview; others argue that the problem with the CPS is a more general underreporting of insurance coverage. Second, although the CPS estimate appears to closely approximate the number of people who are uninsured at a point in time, the survey provides no

information on what fraction of the year people do have coverage.

The Census Bureau added a question to the CPS in March 2000 that should yield a more accurate estimate of the number of uninsured. Previously, people were defined as uninsured throughout the previous calendar year if they responded "no" when asked if they had various types of insurance coverage at any time during that year. The new question, which is designed to verify those responses, specifically asks people who reported no coverage whether in fact they were uninsured. Including that question reduced the CPS estimate of the number of nonelderly people who were uninsured in 1999 from 42.1 million to 39.0 million (or from 17.4 percent to 16.2 percent of the nonelderly population).[1]

The Survey of Income and Program Participation

SIPP is a longitudinal survey in which the same people are interviewed every four months about their insurance status during the previous four months. That shorter reference period should, in principle, yield more accurate data than the CPS provides. SIPP includes a set of questions to determine whether people had various types of

---

1. Based on estimates presented in Charles T. Nelson and Robert J. Mills, "The March CPS Health Insurance Verification Question and Its Effect on Estimates of the Uninsured," Bureau of the Census (August 2001).

Figure A-1.

Distribution of Uninsured Spells That Began Between July 1996 and June 1997, by Duration

(In percent)

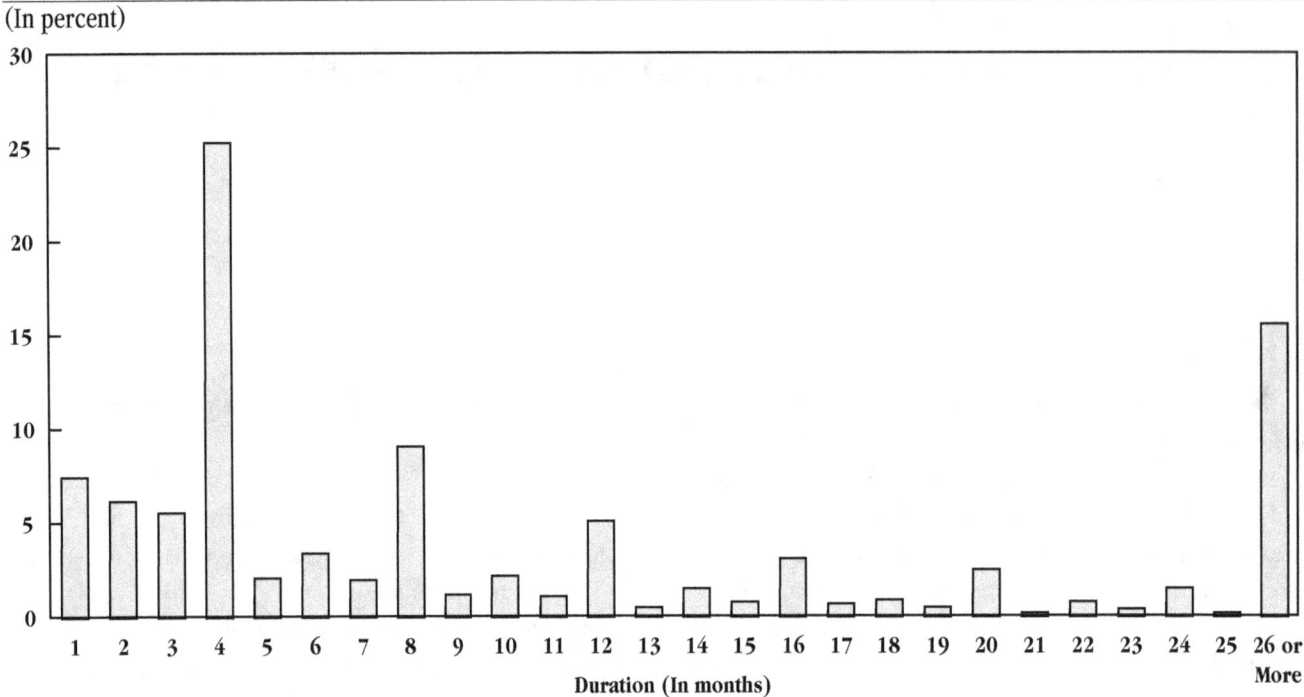

Duration (In months)

Source: Congressional Budget Office based on data from the 1996 panel of the Survey of Income and Program Participation.

Note: The concentration of spells at 26 months includes all spells that lasted at least 26 months. Some of those spells were still in progress at the end of the observation period, so their duration could not be determined.

coverage during each month of the four-month reference period. SIPP does not include a verification question like the one that was added to the March 2000 CPS. Because SIPP data are monthly, researchers are able to compute the percentage of people who were uninsured in a given month, throughout a given year, or at any time during a given year. The Congressional Budget Office's (CBO's) analysis is based on data from the first 11 waves of the 1996 SIPP panel, which provide information on members of the sample from March 1996 through July 1999.

One drawback to SIPP is that its data are released on a less timely basis than are the CPS data. When CBO's analysis was conducted, the most current SIPP data were from the 1996 panel. Second, as with any longitudinal survey, SIPP suffers from sample attrition. That is, some members of the sample drop out over time (because they refuse to continue participating, they move and cannot

be located, and so on). About 25 percent of the original sample in the 1996 SIPP panel was lost through attrition by wave 5, and 34 percent was lost by wave 10. If people who drop out of the sample differ systematically from those who remain with respect to their likelihood of being uninsured or experiencing a long spell without insurance, the SIPP sample may yield biased estimates. To minimize that possibility, CBO's analysis used sampling weights that included an adjustment for the declining number of responses.[2]

_____

2.   The adjustment is constructed by the Census Bureau using information on household size, race, education level, assets, and income sources. However, the adjustment cannot completely account for the ways in which people who drop out of the sample differ from those who remain, because all of the relevant differences between the two groups are not known. Moreover, some attrition may be associated with important changes in a person's circumstances

A third limitation of SIPP is that the data exhibit a "seam effect." Many people appear to report the same insurance status for the entire four-month reference period rather than accurately reporting their status on a month-by-month basis (*see Figure A-1*). About one-quarter of all uninsured spells are reported as lasting four months; other common durations are eight months, 12 months, and so forth. Because of the seam effect, some uninsured spells that are reported as lasting four months, eight months, and so on were actually somewhat shorter or longer. Consequently, CBO's analysis classified spells into categories of reported duration (four months or less, five to 12 months, 13 to 24 months, and more than 24 months).

The Medical Expenditure Panel Survey

As a longitudinal survey, MEPS has the same advantages and disadvantages relative to the Current Population Survey as SIPP does. Like SIPP, MEPS includes a series of questions asking people whether they had various types of insurance in each month of the reference period; the uninsured are defined as those people who report no coverage. Unlike SIPP, in which the reference period is defined as four months for everyone, the reference period in MEPS varies among individuals from three months to five months. The two surveys also differ in their phrasing and sequencing of questions on insurance status.[3]

(such as the loss of employment) that influence the likelihood of being uninsured in the period after having left the sample.

3. For a detailed discussion of the design of SIPP, see Bureau of the Census, *Survey of Income and Program Participation Users' Guide*, 3rd ed. (prepared by Westat in association with Mathematica Policy Research, Inc., 2001). The design of MEPS is described in Steven B. Cohen, *MEPS Methodology Report No. 11*, AHRQ Pub. No. 01-0001 (Rockville, Md: Agency for Healthcare Research and Quality, November 2000).

Those differences may contribute to the different estimates the surveys yield.

In this paper, CBO analyzed data from the MEPS 1999 Full-Year Population Characteristics File, which includes information collected in the third, fourth, and fifth rounds of Panel 3 (which began in 1998) and the first three rounds of Panel 4 (which began in 1999). CBO also analyzed data from the 1998 Full-Year Population Characteristics File to conduct comparisons with 1998 SIPP data.

The National Health Interview Survey

Unlike SIPP and MEPS, NHIS is a cross-sectional survey. Its respondents are not reinterviewed over time to track changes in their insurance status; instead, they are asked to report their status as of the time of the interview and over the previous 12 months. Thus, NHIS yields a point-in-time estimate of the number of people who are uninsured and can, in principle, yield estimates of the number who were ever uninsured during the previous 12 months and the number who were continuously uninsured over that period. However, the Centers for Disease Control and Prevention (CDC), which sponsors the NHIS, reports only the point-in-time estimate.

CBO did not analyze data from the NHIS for this paper because the primary objective was to use longitudinal data from SIPP and MEPS to examine the dynamics of the uninsured. The NHIS point-in-time estimate of the uninsured is included to lend evidence to the argument that the CPS estimate is closer to a point-in-time estimate than a full-year estimate.

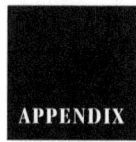
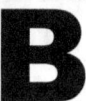

The Consistency of Different Estimates
of the Duration of Uninsured Spells

New uninsured spells are much more likely to be relatively short than are spells in progress at a given point in time. About 45 percent of all new spells last four months or less, compared with only about 8 percent of spells in progress at a given point in time (*see Table 3 on page 9*). In this appendix, the Congressional Budget Office (CBO) demonstrates how the two sets of estimates (those for new spells and spells in progress at a given time) are consistent. CBO also presents estimates of the duration of uninsured spells that were in progress at any time during a one-year period and demonstrates that those estimates are consistent with the observed duration of new spells.

Spells in Progress in a Given Month

CBO used the observed distribution of new uninsured spells to project the distribution of spells in progress at a given point in time.[1] CBO then compared the projections with the actual distribution to gauge their similarity. CBO's method of projecting the duration of spells in progress in a given month was based on the fact that the duration of a spell directly relates to the number of months in which it could have begun. For example, the only one-month spells in progress in a particular month are those that began (and ended) that month, the only two-month spells are those that began in that month or

the prior month, and so on.[2] Likewise, the only 25-month spells in progress in a given month are those that began in that month or in the previous 24 months.

In statistical terms, letting N represent the number of new uninsured spells that began each month over the relevant time period and assuming that N and the distribution of new spells by duration did not change over the period, the total number of spells in progress in a given month (N_p) can be represented as follows:

$$N_p = N\,[.075 + (2)(.062) + (3)(.056) + (4)(.253) + ...]$$

The proportions in the bracketed term reflect the percentage distribution of the duration of new spells shown in Figure A-1 (*see Appendix A*).

The proportion of spells in progress in a given month that are of a particular duration, say three months, can be determined by dividing the projected number of three-

---

1. Although CBO measured spells in progress in March 1998, similar results were obtained for other months.

2. The minimum period of time for which a person's insurance status can be determined in the Survey of Income and Program Participation is one month. Therefore, for analytic purposes, CBO assumed that uninsured spells begin on the first day of a month and end on the last day of a month.

Table B-1.

Projected Distribution of Spells in Progress in a Given Month and a Given Year, by Duration, Based on the Actual Distribution of New Spells

(In percent)

Duration of Uninsured Spells	Actual	Projected[a]
Spells That Began Between July 1996 and June 1997		
Four Months or Less	44.5	n.a.
Five to 12 Months	26.2	n.a.
More Than 12 Months	29.3	n.a.
Spells in Progress in a Given Month[b]		
Four Months or Less	7.9	10.1
Five to 12 Months	13.9	16.4
More Than 12 Months	78.2	73.6
Spells in Progress in a Given Year[b]		
Four Months or Less	22.2	25.4
Five to 12 Months	19.0	20.8
More Than 12 Months	58.8	53.8

Source: Congressional Budget Office based on data from the 1996 panel of the Survey of Income and Program Participation.

Note: n.a. = not applicable.

a.   The projected distributions were computed from the actual distribution of spells that began between July 1996 and June 1997. CBO based its projections on the assumption that the mean duration of new spells that exceed 25 months is 48 months.

b.   The distributions are for spells in progress in March 1998 and from July 1997 through June 1998. Similar estimates were obtained for other time periods.

month spells in progress by the projected total number of spells in progress[3]:

$$(3)(.056) / [.075 + (2)(.062) + (3)(.056) + (4)(.253) + ...]$$

To implement that approach, CBO needed to make an assumption about the mean duration of new spells that exceed 25 months (those spells account for 15.6 percent of all new spells). CBO based its projections on the assumption that the mean duration of such spells is 48 months. That assumption yielded a projected distribution in which 73.6 percent of spells in progress in a given month exceeded 12 months (*see Table B-1*). That figure

is lower than the corresponding 78.2 percent that was estimated directly from the data. To make those two estimates equivalent, CBO would have had to assume that new spells exceeding 25 months had a mean duration of 67 months. If, alternatively, CBO assumed that new spells of more than 25 months lasted, on average, 36 months, the projections would have yielded a distribution in which 69.1 percent of spells in progress in a given month exceeded 12 months.[4]

The projected distribution of spells in progress in a given month is expected to differ from the directly estimated

___

3.   The mean number of spells per month, N, appears in both the numerator and denominator of this expression and therefore cancels out.

4.   A lower-bound estimate was obtained under the extreme (and unrealistic) assumption that all new spells of more than 25 months lasted 26 months. That assumption yielded a projected distribution in which 64.4 percent of the spells in progress in a given month lasted more than 12 months.

distribution for a particular month for two reasons. First, the projections assume that the distribution of the duration of new spells in previous months and the number of new spells that began each month during the observation period remain constant. Departures from that assumption would yield a projected distribution that differed from the actual distribution for a particular month. In addition, long-term chronically uninsured people are underrepresented in the population of new spells but are fully represented in the population of spells in progress in a given month. That discrepancy means that the proportion of long spells in the projected distribution of spells in progress in a given month is lower than in the directly estimated distribution.

CBO's objective in making the projections was not to duplicate the actual distribution of spells in progress in a given month. Instead, the objective was to demonstrate that a flow of new uninsured spells will yield a population of spells in progress in a given month that has a distribution similar to that of the directly estimated distribution.

Spells in Progress in a Given Year

CBO's analysis of uninsured spells showed that 25 percent of the nonelderly population was uninsured at any time in 1998 (*see Table 1 on page 3*). This section of the appendix looks at the duration of those people's uninsured spells and demonstrates that their distribution is consistent with the distribution of the duration of new spells. The analysis focused on people who were uninsured at any time between July 1997 and June 1998 rather than calendar year 1998, in order to provide an adequate time frame for measuring durations.

Fifty-nine percent of the spells experienced by people who were uninsured at any time during the specified 12-month period lasted more than 12 months, whereas 22 percent ended within four months (*see the bottom panel of Table B-1*). CBO obtained those estimates by measuring the total length of spells in progress during the 12-month period, looking backward and forward in time.[5]

People who are uninsured at any time during a particular year are less likely to be experiencing a long uninsured spell than people who are uninsured in a particular month (58.8 percent versus 78.2 percent). As the window used to identify spells under way is extended, the likelihood of capturing short spells increases, because short spells occur much more frequently than longer spells. An even larger proportion of short spells would be captured if the window was extended from, say, 12 months to 24 months.

To illustrate that the estimated distribution of spells in progress in a given year is generally consistent with the distribution of new spells, CBO modified the projection method described earlier. For example, the only one-month spells in progress in a given year are those that began (and ended) within the same month of the 12-month period. Similarly, the only two-month spells are those that began in the month just prior to the year or within the 12-month span. Extending that logic to longer spells, the equation for the number of spells in progress in a given year (N_p) can be expressed as follows:

$$N_p = N\,[(12)(.075) + (13)(.062) + (14)(.056) + (15)(.253) + ...]$$

As before, N is the number of new spells that began per month, and the proportions in the bracketed term reflect the percentage distribution of the duration of new spells.

The proportion of spells in progress in a given year that are of a particular duration, say three months, can be determined as follows:

$$(14)(.056) \,/\, [(12)(.075) + (13)(.062) + (14)(.056) + (15)(.253) + ...]$$

The projections presented in Table B-1 were based on the assumption that new spells exceeding 25 months had a mean duration of 48 months—the same assumption that was used to project spells in progress in a given month. CBO's analysis yielded a projected distribution in which 53.8 percent of spells in progress in a given year were

---

5. For individuals who had more than one uninsured spell during the specified 12-month period, this analysis focused on the first

spell. Through a sensitivity analysis, CBO determined that the decision to focus on the first spell did not affect the results.

longer than 12 months—five percentage points below the 58.8 percent estimated directly from the data. Making those estimates equivalent would have required an assumption that new spells exceeding 25 months had a mean duration of 68 months. If, instead, new spells of more than 25 months were assumed to last 36 months,

on average, the projections would have yielded a distribution in which 49.8 percent of spells in progress in a given year lasted more than 12 months. For the reasons described earlier, however, the projected distributions are not expected to exactly match the actual distributions for a particular year.

www.ingramcontent.com/pod-product-compliance
Lightning Source LLC
Chambersburg PA
CBHW080758290526
45790CB00008B/3504